On Fractures

Hippocrates

TABLE OF CONTENTS

PART 1	1
PART 2	3
PART 3	6
PART 4	9
PART 5	12
PART 6	15
PART 7	17
PART 8	20
PART 9	23
PART 10	25
PART 11	26
PART 12	30
PART 13	31
PART 14	34
PART 15	36
PART 16	38
PART 17	41
PART 18	42
PART 19	44
PART 20	46
PART 21	47
PART 22	48
PART 23	49
PART 24	50
PART 25	52
PART 26	55
PART 27	58
PART 28	61
PART 29	62
PART 30	64
PART 31	67

PART 32	72
PART 33	73
PART 34	75
PART 35	76
PART 36	78
PART 37	80
PART 38	82
PART 39	83
PART 40	84
PART 41	85
PART 42	86
PART 43	88
PART 44	89
PART 45	90
PART 46	91
PART 47	92
PART 48	94

Translated by
Francis Adams

PART 1

In reating fractures and dislocations, the physician must make the extension as straight as possible, for this is the most natural direction. But if it incline to either side, it should rather turn to that of pronation, for there is thus less harm than if it be toward supination. Those, then, who act in such cases without deliberation, for the most part do not fall into any great mistake, for the person who is to have his arm bound, presents it in the proper position from necessity, but physicians who fancy themselves learned in these matters, are they who commit blunders. There is no necessity for much study, then, in order to set a broken arm, and in a word, any ordinary physician can perform it; but I am under the necessity of giving the longer directions on this subject, because I know physicians who have the reputation of being skilled in giving the proper positions to the arm in binding it up, while in reality they are only showing their own ignorance. But many other things in our art are judged of in this manner, for people rather admire what is new, although they do not know whether it be proper or not, than what they are accustomed to, and know already to be proper;

and what is strange, they prefer to what is obvious.I must now state what the mistakes of medical men are, which I wish to unteach, and what instructions I have to give as to the management of the arm; for what I have to say regarding it, will apply to the other bones in the body.

PART 2

The arm, then, for that is the subject we were treating of, was presented in the prone position to be bound, but the physician forced his patient to hold it as the archers do when they project the shoulder, and in this position he bound it up, thinking within himself that he was acting according to Nature, and in proof of this he pointed out that all the bones in the forearm were thus in a straight line, and that the integuments both inside and outside, were also in a straight line, and that the flesh and nerves (tendons?) were thus put in their natural position, and he appealed to what happens in archery, as a proof of this. And so saying, and so doing, he is looked up to as a sage; and yet he forgets that in all the other arts and performances, whether executed whether executed by strength or dexterity, what is reckoned the natural position is not the same, and that in the same piece of work it may happen that the natural position of the right arm is not the same as that of the left. For there is one attitude in throwing the javelin, and another in slinging, another in casting stones, another in boxing, and another in a state of repose. And whatever arts one examines,

it will be found that the natural position of the arms is not the same in each, but that in every case the arms are put into the attitude which suits best with the instrument that is used, and the work to be performed. In practicing archery, no doubt this is the best attitude of the left arm, for gingly-moid extremity of the humerus being fixed in the cavity of the ulna, in this position, throws the bones of the forearm and arm into a line, as if they constituted a single bone, and all flexion at the joint is prevented in this position. It is no doubt certain that the member is thus put into the most unbending and extended position possible, so as not to be overcome or yield when the string is drawn by the right arm, and thus will the archer be enabled to draw the string farthest, and discharge his arrow with the greatest force and rapidity, for arrows thus discharged have the greatest swiftness and force, and are carried to the greatest distances. But there is nothing in common between the binding up of an arm and archery. Moreover, if having thus bound up the arm, the physician direct the patient to keep it thus, he will occasion him greater pain than he had from the wound itself; and thus also, if the physician order him to bend the arm, neither the bones, the nerves, nor the flesh will any longer

be in the same condition, but will be arranged differently, having overcome the bandaging. What use, then, is there of the archer's attitude? And these mistakes, the physician, conceited in his knowledge, would probably not have committed if he had allowed the patient himself to present his arm.

PART 3

But another physician putting the arm into the state of supination, gives orders to extend the arm thus, and bandages it in this position, reckoning it the one according to nature, judging thus from the skin, and also fancying the bones to be thus in their natural position, because the bone which protrudes at the wrist, where the little finger is, appears to be in a line with the bone from which people measure the bone of the forearm. These things he brings forward as proofs that the parts are in their natural state, and he is supposed to speak correctly. But, indeed, if the arm be kept stretched in a supine position, it will become very painful, and this fact any one may ascertain by extending his own arm in this attitude. And also a weaker man grasping with his hands a stronger man whose arm is turned in a supine position, could lead him wherever he chose, and neither, if a man held a sword thus in his hand, could he make any proper use of it, so constrained is this position. And, moreover, if, when a physician has thus bound up the arm, he allow it to remain in the same position, the patient will endure greater pain if he walk about, but considerable, even if he remain at rest. And thus, too, if he shall bend the arm, the muscles and the bones must necessarily assume a different position. But, in addition to other mischief, he is ignorant of these facts regarding the position, that the bone which protrudes at the wrist, close to the little finger, belongs to the forearm, whereas the one at the joint, from which people measure the forearm, is the head of the humerus. He fancies that both these belong to the same bone, and many others are of this opinion. The latter, in fact, is the same part as that which is called the elbow, upon which we sometimes rest, and when he holds the arm thus in a supine position, in the first place the bone appears distorted, and in the next place the tendons which extend from the carpus along the inner side and from the fingers become distorted while the arm has a supine position; for these tendons proceed to the bone of the humerus, from which the forearm is measured. Such, and so many mistakes and marks of ignorance are committed, regarding the natural construction of the arm. But if one will extend a broken arm as I direct, he will turn the bone, situated at the extremity of the little finger, into the straight line, and also the one at the elbow, and the tendons which stretch from the carpus to the extremity of the humerus will be placed in the straight line; and when the arm is suspended in a sling, it will be in the same attitude as that in which it was bound up, and will give no pain to the patient when he walks about, nor when he lies reclined, and will not become fatigued. The man should be so seated that the prominent part of the bone may be turned to the brightest light which is at hand, so that the operator in making the extension, may be at no loss to discover if it be sufficiently straight. The prominence of a broken bone could not escape being detected by the hand of an experienced person, when applied for this purpose, and, moreover, the projecting part is particularly painful to the touch.

PART 4

In cases of fracture in either of the bones of the forearm, it is easier to effect a cure if the upper bone be broken, although it be the thicker one, both because the sound bone is situated below, and forms a support to it, and because the deformity is more easily concealed, there being a thick mass of flesh on the upper side, except near to the wrist. But the lower bone is without a covering of flesh, is not easily concealed, and requires stronger extension. If it is not this bone, but the other which is broken, a more feeble extension proves sufficient, but if both be broken, a more powerful extension is required. In the case of a young person I have known the extension made more strong than was necessary, but in general the extension made is less than what is required. And when they are extended, the physician should apply the palms of the hands, and adjust the fractured parts and then having rubbed the parts with cerate, but not in large quantity so that the bandages may not come off, it is to be bound up in this state, care being taken that the hand be not lower than the elbow, but a little higher, so that the blood do not flow toward the extremity,

but may be determined to the upper part; and then it is to be secured with the bandage, the head of which is to be placed at the fracture, and the bandage should impart firmness to the parts without occasioning strong compression. When you have carried the bandage twice or thrice round at the seat of the fracture, it is to be carried upward, so that the afflux of blood into it may be stopped, and the bandage should terminate there, and the first bandages ought not to be long. The head of the second bandage is also to be placed upon the seat of the fracture, and a single round of it being made there, it is then to be carried downward, and is not to be applied so tight as the other, and there should be greater distances between the turns, so that the bandage may prove sufficient to revert to the spot where the other terminated. The bandages may be rolled to the left hand or to the right, or to whatever side suits best with the position of the fractured arm, or according to the inclination which it may have. Afterward we must place along the arm, compresses, smeared with a little cerate, for thus they occasion less uneasiness, and are more easily arranged. And then we must apply the bandages crossways, sometimes to the right hand, and sometimes to the left, for the most part beginning

below and terminating above, but sometimes commencing above and ending below. The parts which are thinly covered with flesh should be wrapped round with compresses, and inequalities should be made up, not by a number of folds at once, but by degrees. Some slack turns are also to be made around the wrist, to this side and to that. These two bandages are sufficient at first.

PART 5

And these are the signs that the patient has been well treated and properly bandaged: if you ask him if the arm feels tight, and he says it does, but moderately so, and especially about the fracture; and this reply he should make all along, if the bandage be properly applied. And these are symptoms of the bandaging being moderately tight; if for the first day and night he fancies that the tightness does not diminish, but rather increases; and if on the next day there be a soft swelling in the hand, for this is a sign of moderate compression, but at the end of the second day the compression should feel less, and on the third day the bandaging should appear loose. And if any of these symptoms be wanting, you may conclude that the bandaging is slacker than it should be; or if any of these symptoms be in excess, you may infer that the compression is more than moderate; and judging from these, you will apply the next bandages either slacker or tighter. Having removed the bandages on the third day, you must make extension and adjust the fracture, and bind it up again; and if the first bandaging was moderately applied, the second bandaging should be made somewhat tighter. The heads the bandages should be placed on the fractures as in the former case; for, so doing, the humors will be driven to the extremities, whereas if you bandage any other part beforehand, the humors will he forced from it to the seat of the fracture: it is of much importance that this should be properly understood. Thus the bandaging and compression should always commence at the seat of the fracture, and everything else should be conducted on the same principle, so that the farther you proceed from the fracture, the compression should always be the less. The bandages should never be actually loose, but should be smoothly put on. At each dressing the number of bandages should be increased; and the patient, if asked, should answer, that he feels the bandages somewhat tighter than on the former occasion, especially about the fracture, and everything else in proportion; and with respect to the swelling, the pain, and recovery, everything should proceed as after the former dressing. But on the third day the outer bandaging should appear looser. Then having removed the bandages, you should bind it up again, somewhat tighter than before, and with all the bandages which will be required on the occasion, and afterwards one ought

to experience the same train of symptoms as at the former periods of bandaging.

PART 6

When the third day arrives, that is to say, the seventh from the first dressing, if properly done, the swelling in the hand should be not very great; and the part which has been bandaged should be found more slender and less swelled at each time, and on the seventh day the swelling should be quite gone, and the broken bones should be more readily moved, and admit of being easily adjusted. And if these things be so, you should, after setting the fracture, apply the bandages so as to suit the splints, and a little more tight than formerly, unless there be more pain from the swelling in the hand. When you have applied the bandages, you must adjust the splints all around the limb, and secure them secure them with strings so loose as just to keep them in their place, without the application of the splints contributing at all to the compression of the arm. After this the pain and recovery should proceed as in the preceding periods of the bandaging. But if, on the third day, the patient say that the bandaging is loose, you must then fasten the splints, especially at the fracture, but also elsewhere, wherever the bandaging is rather loose than tight. The splint should be thickest where the fracture protrudes, but it should not be much more so than elsewhere. Particular attention should be paid to the line of the arm corresponding to the thumb, so that no splint be laid on it, but upon each side of it, nor in the line of the little finger where the bone is prominent at the wrist, but on each side of it. And if it be found necessary that splints should be applied in these directions at the seat of the fracture, they should be made shorter than the others, so as that they may not reach the bones which are prominent at the wrist, for otherwise there is danger of ulceration, and of the tendons being laid bare. The splints should be adjusted anew every third day, in a very gentle manner, always keeping in mind that the object of the splints is to maintain the lower bandages in their place, and that they are not needed in order to contribute to the compression.

PART 7

If, then, you see that the bones are properly adjusted by the first dressings, and that there is no troublesome pruritus in the part, nor any reason to suspect ulceration, you may allow the arm to remain bandaged in the splints until after the lapse of more than twenty days. The bones of the forearm generally get consolidated in thirty days altogether; but there is nothing precise in this matter, for one constitution differs from another, and one period of life from another. When you remove the bandages, you must pour hot water on the arm and bind it up again, but somewhat slacker, and with fewer bandages than formerly: and again on the third day you undo the bandages, and bind it still more loosely, and with still fewer bandages. And if, while the arm is bound up in the splints, you should at any time suspect that the bones do not lie properly, or if anything about the bandages annoys the patient, you should loose them at the middle of the time, or a little earlier, and apply them again. A diet slightly restricted will be sufficient in those cases in which there was no external wound at first, or when the bone does not protrude; but one should live rather sparingly

until the tenth day, as being now deprived of exercise; and tender articles of food should be used, such as moderately loosen the bowels; but one should abstain altogether from flesh and wine, and then by degrees resume a more nourishing diet. This diet. may be laid down as a just rule in the treatment of fractures, both as to how they should be treated, and what will be the results of a proper plan of treatment; so that one may know, that if things do not turn out thus, there has been some defect or excess in the treatment. And in this simple plan of treatment it is necessary to attend also to the following directions, which some physicians pay little attention to, although, when improperly executed, they are capable of marring the whole process of bandaging: for if both the bones be broken, or the lower one only, and the patient who has got his arm bandaged keep it slung in a shawl, and that the shawl is particularly loose at the fracture, so that the arm is not properly suspended at this end or that, in this case the bone must necessarily be found distorted upwards; whereas, when both bones are thus broken, if the arm recline in the shawl at the wrist and elbow, but the rest of it be not kept up, the bone in this case will be distorted to the lower side. The greater part of the arm and the wrist of

the hand should therefore be equally suspended in a broad soft shawl.

PART 8

When the arm is broken, if one stretch the forearm and adjust it while in this position, the muscle of the arm will be bound while extended; but when the dressing is over, and the patient bends his arm at the elbow, the muscle of the arm will assume a different shape. The following, then, is the most natural plan of setting the arm: having got a piece of wood a cubit or somewhat less in length, like the handles of spades, suspend it by means of a chain fastened to its extremities at both ends; and having seated the man on some high object, the arm is to be brought over, so that the armpit may rest on the piece of wood, and the man can scarcely touch the seat, being almost suspended; then having brought another seat, and placed one or more leather pillows under the arm, so as to keep it a moderate height while it is bent at a right angle, the best plan is to put round the arm a broad and soft skin, or broad shawl, and to hang some great weight to it, so as to produce moderate extension; or otherwise, while the arm is in the position I have described, a strong man is to take hold of it at the elbow and pull it downward. But the physician standing erect, must perform the proper manipulation, having the one foot on some pretty high object, and adjusting the bone with the palms of his hands; and it will readily be adjusted, for the extension is good if properly applied. Then let him bind the arm, commencing at the fracture, and do otherwise as directed above; let him put the same questions and avail himself of the same signs to ascertain whether the arm be moderately tight or not; and every third day let him bind it anew and make it tighter; and on the seventh or ninth day let him bind it up with splints, and leave it so until after the lapse of more than thirty days. And if he suspect that the bone is not lying properly, let him remove the bandages in the interval, and having adjusted the arm, let him bind it up again. The bone of the arm is generally consolidated in forty days. When these are past, the dressing is to be removed, and fewer and slacker bandages applied instead of it. The patient is to be kept on a stricter diet, and for a longer space of time than in the former case; and we must form our judgment of it from the swelling in the hand, looking also to the strength of the patient. This also should be known, that the arm is naturally inclined outward; to this side, therefore, the distortion usually takes place, if not properly treated; but

indeed, all the other bones are usually distorted during treatment for fracture to that side to which they naturally incline. When, therefore, anything of this kind is suspected, the arm is to be encircled in a broad shawl, which is to be carried round the breast, and when the patient goes to rest, a compress of many folds, or some such thing, is to be folded and placed between the elbow and the side, for thus the bending of the bone will be rectified, but care must be taken lest it be inclined too much inwards.

PART 9

The human foot is composed of several small bones like the hand. These bones therefore are scarcely ever broken, unless the skin at the same time be wounded by some sharp and heavy body. The treatment of stich injuries, therefore, will be delivered under the head of wounds. But if any bone be moved from its place, or a joint of the toes be luxated, or any of the bones of the part called the tarsus be displaced, it must be forced back again to its place as described with regard to the hand; and is to be treated with cerate, compresses, and bandages, like the fractures, with the exception of the splints; and is to be secured tightly in the same way, and the bandages renewed on the third day; and the patient thus bandaged should return the same answers as in fractures, as to the bandages feeling tight or slack. All these bones recover perfectly in twenty days, except those that are connected with the bones of the leg, and are in a line with them. It is advantageous to lie in bed during the whole of this time; but the patients, thinking light of the complaint, have not perseverance to do this, and they walk about before they get well; wherefore many of these do

not make a perfect recovery. And often the pain puts them in mind of the injury; and deservedly, for the feet sustain the weight of the whole body. When, therefore, they walk about before they are whole, the joints which have been luxated are cured incompletely; and, on that account, while walking about, they have pains in the leg from time to time.

PART 10

But those bones which are connected with the bones of the leg are larger than the others, and the cure of them when luxuated is more protracted. The mode of treatment then is the same; but we must use more bandages and more splints, and the bandage is to be carried round to this side and to that, and pressure is to be made as in the other cases, particularly at the seat of the luxation, and the first circles of the bandages are to be made there. And at each time the bandages are taken off, much hot water is to be used, for in all injuries at joints the affusion of hot water in large quantity is to be had recourse to. And the same symptoms of compression and relaxation should manifest themselves in the same times, as in the cases formerly treated of, and the subsequent bandagings should be conducted in like manner. These cases get completely well for the most part in forty days, if the patients have resolution to keep their bed; but if not, they are subjected to the complaints formerly described, or still worse.

PART 11

In persons who jumping from any high object pitch upon their heel with great force, the bones are separated, and the veins pour forth their contents, owing to the contusion of the flesh surrounding the bone, and hence a swelling and much pain supervene. For this bone (os calcis) is not a small one, protrudes beyond the line of the leg, and is connected with important veins and tendons; for the back tendon of the leg is inserted into this bone. Such cases are to be treated with cerate, and with compresses and bandages; and hot water is to be used in large quantity; and they require many bandages, which ought to be particularly good and appropriate. And if the patient happen to have a tender skin about the heel, nothing is to be done to it; but if, as some have it, the skin be thick and hardened, it is to be pared down smoothly and thinned, but without wounding it. It is not everybody who can apply the bandage properly in such cases; for if one shall bind the parts, as in other accidents about the ankle, sometimes bringing a fold round the foot and sometimes round the tendon, these turns leave out the heel, which is the seat of the contusion, and thus there is danger that the os calcis may sphacelate; and if this should take place, the impediment may endure for life and also in all the other cases of sphacelus, not proceeding from such a cause as this; as when, from being carelessly allowed to lie in a certain position during confinement to bed, the heel becomes black, or when a serious wound has occurred in the leg and it is long of healing, and is connected with the heel, or when the same thing happens in the thigh, or when in any disease a protracted decubitus takes place on the back, in all such cases the sores are inveterate, troublesome, and frequently break out again, unless particular attention be paid to the cure, along with much rest, as in all the cases attended with sphacelus. And cases of sphacelus connected with this cause, in addition to other inconveniences, are attended with great danger to the whole body. For they are apt to be attended with very acute fevers, of the continual type, accompanied with tremblings, hiccup, aberration of intellect, and which prove fatal within a few days: and there may be lividities of bloody veins, with nausea, and gangrene from pressure; these diseases may occur, besides the sphacelus. Those which have been described are the most violent contusion; but in general the contusions are mild, and no great care is required with regard to the treatment, and yet it must be conducted properly. But when the contusion appears to be severe, we must do as described above, making many turns of the bandage around the heel, sometimes carrying it to the extremity of the foot, sometimes to the middle, and sometimes around the leg; and, in addition, all the surrounding parts are to be bandaged in this direction and that, as formerly described; and the compression should not be made strong, but we should make use of many bandages, and it is better also to administer hellebore the same day or on the morrow; and the bandages should be removed on the third day and reapplied. And these are the symptoms by which we discover whether the case will get worse or not: when the extravasated blood, the lividities, and the surrounding parts become red and hard, there is danger of an exacerbation. But if there be no fever, we must give emetics, as has been said, and administer the other remedies which are applicable when the fever is not of a continual type; but if continual fever be present, we must not give strong medicines, but enjoin abstinence from solid food and soups, and give water for drink, and not allow wine but oxyglyky (a composition from vinegar and honey?). But if the case be not going to get worse, the ecchymosed and livid parts, and those surrounding them become greenish and not hard; for this is a satisfactory proof in all cases of ecchymosis, that they are not to get worse; but when lividity is complicated with hardness, there is danger that the part may become blackened. And we must so manage the foot as that it may be generally raised a little higher than the rest of the body. Such a patient will get well in sixty days if he keep quiet.

PART 12

The leg consists of two bones, of which the one is much more slender than the other at one part, but not much more slender at another. These are connected together at the foot, and form a common epiphysis, but they are not united together along the line of the leg; and at the thigh they are united together and form an epiphysis, and this epiphysis has a diaphysis; but the other bone in a line with the little toe is a little longer. Such is the nature of the bones of the leg.

PART 13

Sometimes the bones connected with the foot are displaced, sometimes both bones with their epiphysis; sometimes the whole epiphysis is slightly moved, and sometimes the other bone. These cases are less troublesome than the same accidents at the wrist, if the patients will have resolution to give them rest. The mode of treatment is the same as that of the other, for the reduction is to be made, as of the other, by means of extension, but greater force is required, as the parts of the body concerned are stronger in this case. But, for the most part, two men will be sufficient, by making extension in opposite directions, but, notwithstanding, if they are not sufficiently strong, it is easy to make more powerful extension in the following way: having fixed in the ground either the nave of a wheel, or any such object, something soft is to be bound round the foot, and then some broad thongs of ox-skin being brought round it, the heads of the thongs are to be fastened to a pestle or any other piece of wood, the end of which is to be inserted into the nave, and it, the pestle, is to be pulled away, while other persons make counter-extension by grasping the shoulders and the ham.

It is also sometimes necessary to secure the upper extremity otherwise; this if you desire to effect, fasten deeply in the ground a round, smooth piece of wood, and place the upper extremity of the piece of wood at the perineum, so that it may prevent the body from yielding to the pulling at the foot, and, moreover, to prevent the leg while stretched, from inclining downward; some person seated at his side should push back the hip, so that the body may not turn round with the pulling, and for this purpose, if you think fit, pieces of wood may be fastened about the armpits on each side, and they are to be stretched by the hands, and thus secured, while another person takes hold of the limb at the knee, and aids in thus making counter-extension. Or thus, if you prefer it: having bound other thongs of leather about the limb, either at the knee, or around the thigh, and having fastened another nave of a wheel in the ground above the head, and adjusted the thongs piece of wood adapted to the nave, extension may thus be made in the opposite direction to the feet. Or if you choose, it may be done thus: instead of the naves, lay a moderate-sized beam under the couch, and then having fastened pieces of wood in this beam, both before and behind the head, make counter-extension by means of thongs, or place

windlasses at this extremity and that, and make extension by means of them. There are many other methods of making extension. But the best thing is, for any physician who practices in a large city, to have prepared a proper wooden machine, with all the mechanical powers applicable in cases of fractures and dislocation, either for making extension, or acting as a lever. For this purpose it will be sufficient to possess a board in length, breadth, and thickness, resembling the quadrangular threshing-boards made of oak.

PART 14

When you have made proper extension, it is easy reduce the joint, for the displaced bone is thus raised into a line with the other. And the bones are to be adjusted with the palms of the hands, pressing upon the projecting bone with the one, and making counter-pressure below the ankle with the other. When you have replaced the bones, you must apply the bandages while the parts are upon the stretch, if you possibly can; but if prevented by the thongs, you must loose them, and make counter-extension until you get the bandages applied. The bandage is to be applied in the manner formerly described, the heads of the bandages being placed on the projecting part, and the first turns made in like manner, and so also with regard to the number of compresses and the compression; and turns of the bandages are to be brought frequently round on this and on that side of the ankle. But this joint must be bound more tight at the first dressing than in the case of the hand. But when you have applied the bandage, you must place the bandaged part somewhat higher than the rest of the body, and in such a position that the foot may hang as little as possible. The attenuation of the body is to be made proportionate to the magnitude of the luxation, for one luxation is to be a small, and another to a great extent. But in general we must reduce more, and for a longer time, in injuries about the legs, than in those about the hands; for the former parts are larger and thicker than the latter, and it is necessary that the body should be kept in a state of rest, and in a recumbent position. There is nothing to prevent or require the limb to be bandaged anew on the third day. And all the treatment otherwise is to be conducted in like manner, as in the preceding cases. And if the patient have resolution to lie quiet, forty days will be sufficient for this purpose, if only the bones be properly reduced, but if he will not lie quiet, he will not be able to use the limb with ease, and he will find it necessary to wear a bandage for a long time. When the bones are not properly replaced, but there has been some defect in this respect, the hip, the thigh, and the leg become wasted, and if the dislocation be inward, the external part of the thigh is wasted, and vice versa. But for the most part the dislocation is inward.

PART 15

And when both bones of the leg are broken without a wound of the skin, stronger extension is required. We may make extension by some of the methods formerly described, provided the bones ride over one another to a considerable degree. But extension by men is also sufficient, and for the most part two strong men will suffice, by making extension and counterextension. Extension must naturally be made straight in a line with the leg and thigh, whether on account of a fracture of the bones of the leg or of the thigh. And in both cases they are to be bandaged while in a state of extension, for the same position does not suit with the leg and the arm. For when the fractured bones of the arm or forearm are bandaged, the forearm is suspended in a sling, and if you bind them up while extended, the figures of the fleshy parts will be changed in bending the arm at the elbow, for the elbow cannot be kept long extended, since persons are not in the custom of keeping the joint long in this form, but in a bent position, and persons who have been wounded in the arm, and are still able to walk about, require to have the arm bent at the elbow-joint. But the leg, both in walking and standing, is habitually extended, either completely or nearly so, and is usually in a depending position from its construction, and in order that it may bear the weight of the rest of the body. Wherefore it readily bears to be extended when necessary, and even when in bed the limb is often in this position. And when wounded, necessity subdues the understanding, since the patients become incapable of raising themselves up, so that they neither think of bending the limb nor of getting up erect, but remain lying in the same position. For these reasons, neither the same position nor the same mode of bandaging applies to the arm and to the leg. If, then, extension by means of men be sufficient, we should not have recourse to any useless contrivances, for it any useless contrivances, for it is absurd to employ mechanical means when not required; but if extension by men be not sufficient, you may use any of the mechanical powers which is suitable. When sufficiently extended, it will be easy to adjust the bones and bring them into their natural position, by straightening and arranging them with the palms of the hand.

PART 16

When the parts are adjusted, you should apply the bandages while the limb is in a stretched position, making the first turns to the right or to the left, as may be most suitable; and the end of the bandage should be placed over the fracture, and the first turns made at that place; and then the bandage should be carried up the leg, as described with regard to the other fractures. But the bandages should be broader and longer, and more numerous, in the case of the leg than in that of the arm. And when it is bandaged it should be laid upon some smooth and soft object, so that it may not be distorted to the one side or the other, and that there may be no protrusion of the bones either forward or backward; for this purpose nothing is more convenient than a cushion, or something similar, either of linen or wool, and not hard; it is to be made hollow along its middle, and placed below the limb. With regard to the canals (gutters?) usually placed below fractured legs, I am at a loss whether to advise that they should be used or not. For they certainly are beneficial, but not to the extent which those who use them suppose. For the canals do not preserve the leg at rest as they suppose; nor, when the rest of the body is turned to the one side or the other, does the canal prevent the leg from following, unless the patient himself pay attention; neither does the canal prevent the limb from being moved without the body to the one side or the other. And a board is an uncomfortable thing to have the limb laid upon, unless something soft be placed above it. But it is a very useful thing in making any subsequent arrangements of the bed and in going to stool. A limb then may be well or ill arranged with or without the canal. But the common people have more confidence, and the surgeon is more likely to escape blame, when the canal is placed under the limb, although it is not secundum artem. For the limb should by all means lie straight upon some level and soft object, since the bandaging must necessarily be overcome by any distortion in the placing of the leg, whenever or to whatever extent it may be inclined. The patient, when bandaged, should return the same answers as formerly stated, for the bandaging should be the same, and the same swellings should arise in the extremities, and the slackening of the bandages in like manner, and the new bandaging on the third day; and the bandaged part should be found reduced in swelling; and the new bandagings should be more tightly put on, and more pieces of cloth should be used; and the bandages should be carried loosely about the foot, unless the wound be near the knee. Extension should be made and the bones adjusted at every new bandaging; for, if properly treated, and if the swelling progress in a suitable manner, the bandaged limb will have become more slender and attenuated, and the bones will be more mobile, and yield more readily to extension. On the seventh, the ninth, or the eleventh day, the splints should be applied as described in treating of the other fractures. Attention should be paid to the position of the splints about the ankles and along the tendon of the foot which runs up the leg. The bones of the leg get consolidated in forty days, if properly treated. But if you suspect that anything is wanting to the proper arrangement of the limb, or dread any ulceration, you should loose the bandages in the interval, and having put everything right, apply them again.

PART 17

But if the other bone (fibula?) of the leg be broken, less powerful extension is required, and yet it must not be neglected, nor be performed slovenly, more especially at the first bandaging. For in all cases of fracture this object should be attained then as quickly as possible. For when the bandage is applied tight while the bones are not properly arranged, the properly arranged, the part becomes more painful. The treatment otherwise is the same.

PART 18

Of the bones of the leg, the inner one, called the tibia, is the more troublesome to manage, and requires the greater extension; and if the broken bones are not properly arranged, it is impossible to conceal the distortion, for the bone is exposed and wholly uncovered with flesh; and it is much longer before patients can walk on the leg when this bone is broken. But if the outer bone be broken, it causes much less trouble, and the deformity, when the bones are not properly set, is much more easily concealed, the bone being well covered with flesh; and the patients speedily get on foot, for it is the inner bone of the leg which supports the most of the weight of the body. For along with the thigh, as being in a line with weight thrown upon the thigh, the inner bone has more work to sustain; inasmuch as it is the head of the thigh-bone which sustains the upper part of the body, and it is on the inner and not on the outer side of the thigh, being in a line with the tibia; and the other half of the body approximates more to this line than to the external one; and at the same time the inner bone is larger than the outer, as in the forearm the bone in the line of the little finger is the slenderer and longer. But in the joint of the inferior extremity, the disposition of the longer bone is not alike, for the elbow and the ham are bent differently. For these reasons when the external bone is broken, the patients can soon walk about; but in fractures of the inner, it is a long time before they can walk.

PART 19

When the thighbone is broken, particular pains should be taken with regard to the extension that it may not be insufficient, for when excessive, no great harm results from it. For, if one should bandage a limb while the extremities of the bone are separated to a distance from one another by the force of the extension, the bandaging will not keep them separate, and so the bones will come together again as soon as the persons stretching it let go their hold; for the fleshy parts (muscles?) being thick and strong, are more powerful than the bandaging, instead of being less so. In the case then which we are now treating of, nothing should be omitted in order that the parts may be properly distended and put in a straight line; for it is a great disgrace and an injury to exhibit a shortened thigh. For the arm, when shortened, might be concealed, and the mistake would not be great; but a shortened thighbone would exhibit the man maimed. For when the sound limb is placed beside it, being longer than the other, it exposes the mistake, and therefore it would be to the advantage of a person who would be improperly treated that both his legs should be broken, rather than either of them; for in this case the one would be of the same length as the other. When, then, proper extension has been made, you must adjust the parts with the palms of the hands, and bandage the limb in the manner formerly described, placing the hands of the bandages as was directed, and making the turns upward. And the patient should return the same answers to the same questions as formerly, should be pained and recover in like manner, and should have the bandaging renewed in the same way; and the application of the splints should be the same. The thighbone is consolidated in forty days.

PART 20

But this also should be known, that the thighbone is curved rather to the outside than to the inside, and rather forward than backward; when not properly treated, then, the distortions are in these directions; and the bone is least covered with flesh at the same parts, so that the distortion cannot be concealed. If, therefore, you suspect anything of this kind, you should have recourse to the mechanical contrivances recommended in distortion of the arm. And a few turns of the bandage should be brought round by the hip and the loins, so that the groin and the articulation near the perineum may be included in the bandage; and moreover, it is expedient that the extremities of the splints should not do mischief by being placed on parts not covered with the bandages. The splints, in fact, should be carefully kept off the naked parts at both ends; and the arrangement of them should be so managed, as that they may not be placed on the natural protuberances of the bone at the knee-joint, nor on the tendon which is situated there.

PART 21

The swellings which arise in the ham, at the foot, or in any other part from the pressure, should be well wrapped in unscoured and carded wool, washed with wine and oil, and anointed with cerate, before bandaging; and if the splints give pain they should be slackened. You may sooner reduce the swellings, by laying aside the splints, and applying plenty of bandages to them, beginning from below and rolling upward; for thus the swellings will be most speedily reduced, and the humors be propelled to the parts above the former bandages. But this form of bandaging must not be used unless there be danger of vesications or blackening in the swelling, and nothing of the kind occurs unless the fracture be bound too tight, or unless the limb be allowed to hang, or it be rubbed with the hand, or some other thing of an irritant nature be applied to the skin.

PART 22

More injury than good results from placing below the thigh a canal which does not pass farther down than the ham, for it neither prevents the body nor the leg from being moved without the thigh. And it creates uneasiness by being brought down to the ham, and has a tendency to produce what of all things should be avoided, namely, flexion at the knee, for this completely disturbs the bandages; and when the thigh and leg are bandaged, if one bend the limb at the knee, the muscles necessarily assume another shape, and the broken bones are also necessarily moved. Every endeavor then should be made to keep the ham extended. But it appears to me, that a canal which embraces the limb from the nates to the foot is of use. And moreover, a shawl should be put loosely round at the ham, along with the canal, as children are swathed in bed; and then, if the thighbone gets displaced either upward or to the side, it can be more easily kept in position by this means along with the canal. The canal then should be made so as to extend all along the limb or not used at all.

PART 23

The extremity of the heel should be particularly attended to, so that it may be properly laid, both in fractures of the leg and of the thigh. For if the foot be placed in a dependent position, while the rest of the body is supported, the limb must present a curved appearance at the forepart of the leg; and if the heel be placed higher than is proper, and if the rest of the leg be rather too low, the bone at the forepart of the leg must present a hollow, more especially if the heel of the patient be naturally large. But all the bones get consolidated more slowly, if not laid properly, and if not kept steady in the same position, and in this case the callus is more feeble.

PART 24

These things relate to cases in which there is fracture of the bones without protrusion of the same or wound of any other kind. In those cases in which the bones are simply broken across, and are not comminuted, but protrude, if reduced the same day or next, and secured in their place, and if there be no reason to anticipate that any splintered bones will come away; and in those in which the broken bones do not protrude, nor is the mode of fracture such that there is reason to expect the splinters will come out, some physicians heal the sores in a way which neither does much good nor harm, by means of a cleansing application, applying pitch ointment, or some of the dressings for fresh wounds, or anything else which they are accustomed to do, and binding above them compresses wetted with wine, or greasy wool, or something else of the like nature. And when the wounds become clean and are new healed, they endeavor to bind up the limb with plenty of bandages, and keep it straight with treatment does some good, and never much harm. The bones, however, can never be equally well restored to their place, but the part is a little more

swelled than it should be; and the limb will be somewhat shortened, provided both bones either of the leg or forearm have been fractured.

PART 25

There are others who treat such cases at first with bandages, applying them on both sides of the seat of the injury, but omit them there, and leave the wound uncovered, and afterward they apply to the wound some cleansing medicine, and complete the dressing with compresses dipped in wine and greasy wool. This plan of treatment is bad, and it is clear that those who adopt this mode of practice are guilty of great mistakes in other cases of fracture as well as these. For it is a most important consideration to know in what manner the head of the bandage should be placed and at what part the greatest pressure should be, and what benefits would result from applying the end of the bandage and the pressure at the proper place, and what mischiefs would result from applying the head of the bandage and the pressure otherwise than at the proper place. Wherefore it has been stated in the preceding part of the work what are the results of either; and the practice of medicine bears witness to the truth of it, for in a person thus bandaged, a swelling must necessarily arise on the wound. For, if even a sound piece of skin were bandaged on either side, and a part were left in the middle, the part thus left unbandaged would become most swelled, and would assume a bad color; how then could it be that a wound would not suffer in like manner? The wound then must necessarily become discolored and its lips everted, the discharge will be ichorous and without pus, and the bones, which should not have got into a state of necrosis, exfoliate; and the wound gets into a throbbing and inflamed condition. And they are obliged to apply a cataplasm on account of the swelling, but this is an unsuitable application to parts which are bandaged on both sides, for a useless load is added to the throbbing which formerly existed in it. At last they loose the bandages when matters get very serious, and conduct the rest of the treatment without bandaging; and notwithstanding, if they meet with another case of the same description, they treat it in the same manner, for they do not think that the application of the bandages on both sides, and the exposure of the wound are the cause of what happened, but some other untoward circumstance. Wherefore I would not have written so much on this subject, if I had not well known that this mode of bandaging is unsuitable, and yet that many conduct the treatment in this way, whose mistake it is of vital importance to correct, while what is here said is a proof, that what was formerly written as to the circumstances under which bandages should be tightly applied to fractures or otherwise has been correctly written.

PART 26

As a general rule it may be said, that in those cases in which a separation of bone is not expected, the same treatment should be applied as when the fractures are not complicated with an external wound; for the extension, adjustment of the bones, and the bandaging, are to be conducted in the same manner. To the wound itself a cerate mixed with pitch is to be applied, a thin folded compress is to be bound upon it, and the parts around are to be anointed with white cerate. The cloths for bandages and the other things should be torn broader than in cases in which there is no wound, and the first turn of the bandage should be a good deal broader than the wound. For a narrower bandage than the wound binds the wound like a girdle, which is not proper, or the first turn should comprehend the whole wound, and the bandaging should extend beyond it on both sides. The bandage then should be put on in the direction of the wound, and should be not quite so tight as when there is no wound, but the bandage should be otherwise applied in the manner described above. The bandages should be of a soft consistence, and more especially so in such cases than in those not complicated with a wound. The number of bandages should not be smaller, but rather greater than those formerly described. When applied, the patient should have the feeling of the parts being properly secured, but not too tight, and in particular he should be able to say that they are firm about the wound. And the intervals of time during which the parts seem to be properly adjusted, and those in which they get loose, should be the same as those formerly described. The bandages should be renewed on the third day, and the after treatment conducted in the same manner as formerly described, except that in the latter case the compression should be somewhat less than in the former. And if matters go on properly, the parts about the wound should be found at every dressing always more and more free of swelling, and the swelling should have subsided on the whole part comprehended by the bandages. And the suppurations will take place more speedily than in the case of wounds treated otherwise; and the pieces of flesh in the wound which have become black and dead, will sooner separate and fall off under this plan of treatment than any other, and the sore will come more quickly to cicatrization when thus treated than otherwise. The reason of all this is, that the parts in which the wound is situated, and the surrounding parts, are kept free of swelling. In all other respects the treatment is to be conducted as in cases of fracture without a wound of the integuments. Splints should not be applied. On this account the bandages should be more numerous than in the former case, both because they must be put on less tight, and because the splints are later of being applied. But if you do apply the splints, they should not be applied along the wound, and they are to be put on in a loose manner, especial care being taken that there may be no great compression from the splints. This direction has been formerly given. And the diet should be more restricted, and for a longer period, in those cases in which there is a wound at the commencement, and when the bones protrude through the skin; and, in a word, the greater the wound, the more severe and protracted should the regimen be.

PART 27

The treatment of the sores is the same in those cases of fracture in which there was no wound of the skin at first, but one has formed in the course of treatment, owing to the pressure of the splints occasioned by the bandages, or from any other cause. In such cases it is ascertained that there is an ulcer, by the pain and the throbbing; and the swelling in the extremities becomes harder than usual, and if you apply your finger the redness disappears, but speedily returns. If you suspect anything of the kind you must loose the dressing, if there be any itching below the under-bandages, or in any other part that is bandaged, and used a pitched cerate instead of the other. If there be nothing of that, but if the ulcer be found in an irritable state, being very black and foul, and the fleshy parts about to suppurate, and the tendons to slough away, in these cases no part is to be exposed to the air, nor is anything to be apprehended from these suppurations, but the treatment is to be conducted in the same manner as in those cases in which there was an external wound at first. You must begin to apply the bandages loosely at the swelling in the extremities, and then gradually proceed upward with the bandaging, so that it may be tight at no place, but particularly firm at the sore, and less so elsewhere. The first bandages should be clean and not narrow, and the number of bandages should be as great as in those cases in which the splints were used, or somewhat fewer. To the sore itself a compress, anointed with white cerate, will be sufficient, for if a piece of flesh or nerve (tendon?) become black, it will fall off; for such sores are not to be treated with acrid, but with emollient applications, like burns. The bandages are to be renewed every third day, and no splints are to be applied, but rest is to be more rigidly maintained than in the former cases, along with a restricted diet. It should be known, that if any piece of flesh or tendon be to come away, the mischief will spread much less, and the parts will much more speedily drop off, and the swelling in the surrounding parts will much more completely subside, under this treatment, than if any of the cleansing applications be put upon the sore. And if any part that is to come away shall fall off, the part will incarnate sooner when thus treated than otherwise, and will more speedily cicatrize. Such are the good effects of knowing how a bandage can be well and moderately applied. But a proper

position, the other parts of the regimen, and suitable bandages cooperate.

PART 28

If you are deceived with regard to a recent wound, supposing there will be no exfoliation of the bones, while they are on the eve of coming out of the sore, you must not hesitate to adopt this mode of treatment; for no great mischief will result, provided you have the necessary dexterity to apply the bandages well and without doing any harm. And this is a symptom of an exfoliation of bone being about to take place under this mode of treatment; pus runs copiously from the sore, and appears striving to make its escape. The bandage must be renewed more frequently on account of the discharge, since otherwise fevers come on; if the sore and surrounding parts be compressed by the bandages they become wasted. Cases complicated with the exfoliation of very small bones, do not require any change of treatment, only the bandages should be put on more loosely, so that the discharge of pus may not be intercepted, but left free, and the dressings are to be frequently renewed until the bone exfoliate, and the splints should not be applied until then.

PART 29

Those cases in which the exfoliation of a larger piece of bone is expected, whether you discover this at the commencement, or perceive subsequently that it is to happen, no longer require the same mode of treatment, only that the extension and arrangement of the parts are to be performed in a manner that has been described; but having formed double compresses, not less than half a fathom in breadth (being guided in this by the nature of the wound), and considerably shorter than what would be required to go twice round the part that is wounded, but considerably longer than to go once round, and in number what will be sufficient, these are to be dipped in a black austere wine; and beginning at the middle, as is done in applying the double-headed bandage, you are to wrap the part around and proceed crossing the heads in the form of the bandage called "ascia." These things are to be done at the wound, and on both sides of it; and there must be no compression, but they are to be laid on so as to give support to the wound. And on the wound itself is to be applied the pitched cerate, or one of the applications to recent wounds, or any other

medicine which will suit with the embrocation. And if it be the summer season, the compresses are to be frequently damped with wine; but if the winter season, plenty of greasy wool, moistened with wine and oil, should be applied. And a goat's skin should be spread below, so as to carry off the fluids which run from the wound; these must be guarded against, and it should be kept in mind, that parts which remain long in the same position are subject to excoriations which are difficult to cure.

PART 30

In such cases as do not admit of bandaging according to any of the methods which have been described, or which will be described, great pains should be taken that the fractured part of the body be laid in a right position, and attention should be paid that it may incline upward rather than downward. But if one would wish to do the thing well and dexterously, it is proper to have recourse to some mechanical contrivance, in order that the fractured part of the body may undergo proper and not violent extension; and this means is particularly applicable in fractures of the leg. There are certain physicians who, in all fractures of the leg, whether bandages be applied or not, fasten the sole of the foot to the couch, or to some other piece of wood which they have fixed in the ground near the couch. These persons thus do all sorts of mischief but no good; for it contributes nothing to the extension that the foot is thus bound, as the rest of the body will no less sink down to the foot, and thus the limb will no longer be stretched, neither will it do any good toward keeping the limb in a proper position, but will do harm, for when the rest of the body is turned to this side or that, the bandaging will not prevent the foot and the bones belonging to it from following the rest of the body. For if it had not been bound it would have been less distorted, as it would have been the less prevented from following the motion of the rest of the body.But one should sew two balls of Egyptian leather, such as are worn by persons confined for a length of time in large shackles, and the balls the balls should have coats on each side, deeper toward the wound, but shorter toward the joints; and the balls should be well stuffed and soft, and fit well, the one above the ankles, and the other below the knee. Sideways it should have below two appendages, either of a single or double thong, and short, like loops, the one set being placed on either side of the ankle, and the other on the knee. And the other upper ball should have others of the same kind in the same line. Then taking four rods, made of the cornel tree, of equal length, and of the thickness of a finger, and of such length that when bent they will admit of being adjusted to the appendages, care should be taken that the extremities of the rods bear not upon the skin, but on the extremities of the balls. There should be three sets of rods, or more, one set a little longer than another, and another a little shorter and smaller, so that they may produce greater or less distention, if required.Either of these sets of rods should be placed on this side and that of the ankles. If these things be properly contrived, they should occasion a proper and equable extension in a straight line, without giving any pain to the wound; for the pressure, if there is any, should be thrown at the foot and the thigh. And the rods are commodiously arranged on either side of the ankles, so as not to interfere with the position of the limb; and the wound is easily examined and easily arranged. And, if thought proper, there is nothing to prevent the two upper rods from being fastened to one another; and if any light covering be thrown over the limb, it will thus be kept off from the wound. If, then, the balls be well made, handsome, soft, and newly stitched, and if the extension by the rods be properly managed, as has been already described, this is an excellent contrivance; but if any of them do not fit properly, it does more harm than good.And all other mechanical contrivances should either be properly done, or not be had recourse to at all, for it is a disgraceful and awkward thing to use mechanical means in an unmechanical way.

PART 31

Moreover, the greater part of physicians treat fractures, both with and without an external wound, during the first days, by means of unwashed wool, and there does not appear to be anything improper in this. It is very excusable for those who are called upon to treat newly-received accidents of this kind, and who have no cloth for bandages at hand, to do them up with wool; for, except cloth for bandages, one could not have anything better than wool in such cases; but a good deal should be used for this purpose, and it should be well carded and not rough, for in small quantity and of a bad quality it has little power. But those who approve of binding up the limb with wool for a day or two, and on the third and fourth apply bandages, and make the greatest compression and extension at that period, such persons show themselves to be ignorant of the most important principles of medicine; for, in a word, at no time is it so little proper to disturb all kinds of wounds as on the third and fourth day; and all sort of probing should be avoided on these days in whatever other injuries are attended with irritation. For, generally, the third and fourth day in most cases of wounds, are those which give rise to exacerbations, whether the tendency be to inflammation, to a foul condition of the sore, or to fevers. And if any piece of information be particularly valuable this is; to which of the most important cases in medicine does it not apply? and that not only in wounds but in many other diseases, unless one should call all other diseases wounds. And this doctrine is not devoid of a certain degree of plausibility, for they are allied to one another in many respects. But those who maintain that wool should be used until after the first seven days, and then that the parts should be extended and adjusted, and secured with bandages, would appear not to be equally devoid of proper judgment, for the proper judgment, for the most dangerous season for inflammation is then past, and the bones being loose can be easily set after the lapse of these days. But still this mode of treatment is far inferior to that with bandages from the commencement; for, the latter method exhibits the patient on the seventh day free from inflammation, and ready for complete bandaging with splints; while the former method is far behind in this respect, and is attended with many other bad effects which it would be tedious to describe.

31a. In those cases of fracture in which the bones protrude and cannot be restored to their place, the following mode of reduction may be practiced:– Some small pieces of iron are to be prepared like the levers which the cutters of stone make use of, one being rather broader and another narrower; and there should be three of them at least, and still more, so that you may use those that suit best; and then, along with extension, we must use these as levers, applying the under surface of the piece of iron to the under fragment of the bone, and the upper surface to the upper bone; and, in a word, we must operate powerfully with the lever as we would do upon a stone or a piece of wood. The pieces of iron should be as strong as possible, so that they may not bend. This is a powerful assistance, provided the pieces of iron be suitable, and one use them properly as levers. Of all the mechanical instruments used by men, the most powerful are these three, the axis in peritrochio, the lever, and the wedge. Without these, one or all, men could not perform any of their works which require great force. Wherefore, reduction with the lever is not to be despised, for the bones will be reduced in this way, or not at all. But if the upper fragment which rides over the other does not furnish a suitable point of support a suitable point of support for the lever, but the protruding part is sharp, you must scoop out of the bone what will furnish a proper place for the lever to rest on. The lever, along with extension, may be had recourse to on the day of the accident, or the accident, or next day, but by no means on the third, the fourth, and the fifth. For if the limb is disturbed on these days, and yet the fractured bones not reduced, inflammation will be excited, and this no less if they are reduced; for convulsions are more apt to occur if reduction take place, than if the attempt should fail. These facts should be well known, for if convulsions should come on when reduction is effected, there effected, there is little hope of recovery; but it is of use to displace the bones again if this can be done with out trouble. For it is not at the time when the parts are in a particularly relaxed condition that convulsions and tetanus are apt to supervene, but when they are more than usually tense. In the case we are now treating of, we should not disturb the limb on the aforesaid days, but strive to keep the wound as free from inflammation as possible, and especially encourage suppuration in it. But when seven days have elapsed, or rather more, if there be no fever, and if the wound be not inflamed, then there will be

less to prevent an attempt at reduction, if you hope to succeed; but otherwise you need not take and give trouble in vain.

PART 32

When you have reduced the bones to their place, the modes of treatment, whether you expect the bones to exfoliate or not, have been already described. All those cases in which an exfoliation of bone is expected, should be treated by the method of bandaging with cloths, beginning for the most part at the middle of the bandage, as is done with the double-headed bandage; but particular attention should be paid to the shape of the wound, so that its lips may gape or be distorted as little as possible under the bandage. Sometimes the turns of the bandage have to be made to the right, and sometimes to the left, and sometimes a double-headed bandage is to be used.

PART 33

It should be known that bones, which it has been found impossible to reduce, as well as those which are wholly denuded of flesh, will become detached. In some cases the upper part of the bone is laid bare, and in others the flesh dies all around; and, from a sore of long standing, certain of the bones become carious, and some not, some more, and some less; and in some the small, and in others the large bones. From what has been said it will be seen, that it is impossible to tell in one word when the bones will separate. Some come away more quickly, owing to their smallness, and some from being merely fixed at the point; and some, from pieces not separating, but merely exfoliating, become dried up and putrid; and besides, different modes of treatment have different effects. For the most part, the bones separate most quickly in those cases in which suppuration takes place most quickly, and when new flesh is most quickly formed, and is particularly sound, for the flesh which grows up below in the wound generally elevates the pieces of bone. It will be well if the whole circle of the bone separate in forty days; for in some cases it is protracted to sixty days, and in some to more; for the more porous pieces of bone separate more quickly, but the more solid come away more slowly; but the other smaller splinters in much less time, and others otherwise. A portion of bone which protrudes should be sawn off for the following reasons: if it cannot be reduced, and if it appears sons: that only a small piece is required in order that it may get back into its place; and if it be such that it can be taken out, and if it occasions inconvenience and irritates any part of the flesh, and prevents the limb from being properly laid, and if, moreover, it be denuded of flesh, such a piece of bone should be taken off. With regard to the others, it is not of much consequence whether they be sawed off or not. For it should be known for certain, that such bones as are completely deprived of flesh, and have become dried, all separate completely. Those which are about to exfollate should not be sawn off. Those that will separate completely must be judged of from the symptoms that have been laid down.

PART 34

Such cases are to be treated with compresses and vinous applications, as formerly laid down regarding bones which will separate. We must avoid wetting it at the beginning with anything cold; for there is danger of febrile rigors, and also of convulsions; for convulsions are induced by cold things, and also sometimes by wounds. It is proper to know that the members are necessarily shortened in those cases in which the bones have been broken, and have healed the one across the other, and in those cases in which the whole circle of the bone has become detached.

PART 35

Those cases in which the bone of the thigh, or of the arm, protrudes, do not easily recover. For the bones are large, and contain much marrow; and many important nerves, muscles, and veins are wounded at the same time. And if you reduce them, convulsions usually supervene; and, if not reduced, acute bilious fevers come on, with singultus and mortification. The chances of recovery are not fewer in those cases in which the parts have not been reduced, nor any attempts made at reduction. Still more recover in those cases in which the lower, than those in which the upper part of the bone protrudes; and some will recover when reduction has been made, but very rarely indeed.For modes of treatment and peculiarity of constitution make a great difference as to the capability of enduring such an injury. And it makes a great difference if the bones of the arm and of the thigh protrude to the inside; for there are many and important vessels situated there, some of which, if wounded, will prove fatal; there are such also on the outside, but of less importance. In wounds of this sort, then, one ought not to be ignorant of the dangers, and should prognosticate them in due time. But if you are compelled to have recourse to reduction, and hope to succeed, and if the bones do not cross one another much, and if the muscles are not contracted (for they usually are contracted), the lever in such cases may be advantageously employed.

PART 36

Having effected the reduction, you must give an emollient draught of hellebore the same day, provided it has been reduced on the day of the accident, but otherwise it should not be attempted. The wound should be treated with the same things as are used in fractures of the bones of the head, and nothing cold should be applied; the patient should be restricted from food altogether, and if naturally of a bilious constitution, he should have for a diet a little fragrant oxyglyky sprinkled on water; but if he is not bilious, he should have water for drink; and if fever of the continual type come on, he is to be confined to this regimen for fourteen days at least, but if he be free of fever, for only seven days, and then you must bring him back by degrees to a common diet. To those cases in which the bones have not been reduced, a similar course of medicine should be administered, along with the same treatment of the sores and regimen; and in like manner the suspended part of the body should not be stretched, but should rather be contracted, so as to relax the parts about the wound. The separation of the bones is protracted, as also was formerly stated. But one should

try to escape from such cases, provided one can do so honourably, for the hopes of recovery are small, and the dangers many; and if the physician do not reduce the fractured bones he will be looked upon as upon as unskillful, while by reducing them he will bring the patient nearer to death than to recovery.

PART 37

Luxations and subluxations at the knee are much milder accidents than subluxations and luxations at the elbow. For the knee-joint, in proportion to its size, is more compact than that of the arm, and has a more even conformation, and is rounded, while the joint of the arm is large, and has many cavities. And in addition, the bones of the leg are nearly of the same length, for the external one overtops the other to so small an extent as hardly to deserve being mentioned, and therefore affords no great resistance, although the external nerve (ligament?) at the ham arises from it; but the bones of the forearm are unequal, and the shorter is considerably thicker than the other, and the more slender (ulna?) protrudes, and passes up above the joint, and to it (the olecranon?) are attached the nerves (ligaments?) which go downward to the junction of the bones; and the slender bone (ulna?) has more to do with the insertion of the ligaments in the arm than the thick bone (radius?). The configuration then of the articulations, and of the bones of the elbow, is such as I have described. Owing to their configuration, the bones at the knee are indeed frequently dislocated, but they are easily reduced, for no great inflammation follows, nor any constriction of the joint. They are displaced for the most part to the inside, sometimes to the outside, and occasionally into the ham. The reduction in all these cases is not difficult, but in the dislocations inward and outward, the patient should be placed on a low seat, and the thigh should be elevated, but not much. Moderate extension for the most part sufficeth, extension being made at the leg, and counter-extension at the thigh.

PART 38

Dislocations at the elbow are more troublesome than those at the knee, and, owing to the inflammation which comes on, and the configuration of the joint, are more difficult to reduce if the bones are not immediately replaced. For the bones at the elbow are less subject to dislocation than those of the knee, but are more difficult to reduce and keep in their position, and are more apt to become inflamed and ankylosed.

PART 39

For the most part the displacements of these bones are small, sometimes toward the ribs, and sometimes to the outside; and the whole articulation is not displaced, but that part of the humerus remains in place which is articulated with the cavity of the bone of the forearm that has a protuberance (ulna?). Such dislocations, to whatever side, are easily reduced, and the extension is to be made in the line of the arm, one person making extension at the wrist, and another grasping the armpit, while a third, applying the palm of his hand to the part of the joint which is displaced, pushes it inward ward, and at the same time makes counterpressure on the opposite side near the joint with the other hand.

PART 40

The end of the humerus at the, elbow gets displaced (subluxated?) by leaving the cavity of the ulna. Such luxations readily yield to reduction, if applied before the parts get inflamed. The displacement for the most part is to the inside, but sometimes to the outside, and they are readily recognized by the shape of the limb. And often such luxations are reduced without any powerful extension. In dislocations inward, the joint is to be pushed into its place, while the forearm is brought round to a state of pronation. Such are most of the dislocations at the elbow.

PART 41

But if the articular extremity of the humerus be carried to either side above the bone of the forearm, which is prominent, into the hollow of the arm (?), this rarely happens; but if it does happen, extension in the straight line is not so proper under such circumstances; for in such a mode of extension, the process of the ulna (olecranon?) prevents the bone of the arm (humerus?) from passing over it. In dislocations of this kind, extension should be made in the manner described when treating of the bandaging of fractured bones of the arm, extension being made upward at the armpit, while the parts at the elbow are pushed downward, for in this manner can the humerus be most readily raised above its cavity; and when so raised, the reduction is easy with the palms of the hand, the one being applied so as to make pressure on the protuberant part of the arm, and the other making counter-pressure, so as to push the bone of the forearm into the joint. This method answers with both cases. And perhaps this is the most suitable mode of reduction in such a case of dislocation. The parts may be reduced by extension in a straight line, but less readily than thus.

PART 42

If the arm be dislocated forward\emdash this rarely happens, indeed, but what would a sudden shock not displace? for many other things are removed from their proper place, notwithstanding a great obstacle,\emdash in such a violent displacement the part (olecranon?) which passes above the prominent part of the bones is large, and the stretching of the nerves (ligaments?) is intense; and yet the parts have been so dislocated in certain cases. The following is the symptom of such a displacement: the arm cannot be bent in the least degree at the elbow, and upon feeling the joint the nature of the accident becomes obvious. If, then, it is not speedily reduced, strong and violent inflammation, attended with fever, will come on, but if one happen to be on the spot at the time it is easily reduced. A piece of hard linen cloth (or a piece of hard linen, not very large, rolled up in a ball, will be sufficient) is to be placed across the bend of the elbow, and the arm is then to be suddenly bent at the elbow, and the hand brought up to the shoulder. This mode of reduction is sufficient in such displacements; and extension in the straight line can rectify this manner of dislocation, but we must use at the same time the palms of the hands, applying the one to the projecting part of the humerus at the bend of the arm for the purpose of pushing it back, and applying the other below to the sharp extremity of the elbow, to make counter-pressure, and incline the parts into the straight line. And one may use with advantage in this form of dislocation the method of extension formerly described, for the application of the bandages in the case of fracture of the arm; but when extension is made, the parts are to be adjusted, as has been also described above.

PART 43

But if the arm be dislocated backward (but this very rarely happens, and it is the most painful of all, and the most subject to bilious fevers of the continual type, which prove fatal in the course of a few days), in such a case the patient cannot extend the arm. If you are quickly present, by forcible extension the parts may return to their place of their own accord; but if fever have previously come on, you must no longer attempt reduction, for the pain will be rendered more intense by any such violent attempt. In a word, no joint whatever should be reduced during the prevalence of fever, and least of all the elbow-joint.

PART 44

There are also other troublesome injuries connected with the elbow-joint; for example, the thicker bone (radius?) is sometime partially displaced from the other, and the patient can neither perform extension nor flexion properly. This accident becomes obvious upon examination with the hand at the bend of the arm near the division of the vein that runs up the muscle. In such a case it is not easy to reduce the parts to their natural state, nor is it easy, in the separation of any two bones united by symphysis, to restore them to their natural state, for there will necessarily be a swelling at the seat of the diastasis. The method of bandaging a joint has been already described in treating of the application of bandages to the ankle.

PART 45

In certain cases the process of the ulna (olecranon?) behind the humerus is broken; sometimes its cartilaginous part, which gives origin to the posterior tendon of the arm, and sometimes its fore part, at the base of the anterior coronoid process; and when this displacement takes place, it is apt to be attended with malignant fever. The joint, however, remains in place, for its whole base protrudes at that point. But when the displacement takes place where its head overtops the arm, the joint becomes looser if the bone be fairly broken across. To speak in general terms, all cases of fractured bones are less dangerous than those in which the bones are not broken, but the veins and important nerves (tendons?) situated in these places are contused; for the risk of death is more immediate in the latter class of cases than in the former, if continual fever come on. But fractures of this nature seldom occur.

PART 46

It sometimes happens that the head of the humerus is fractured at its epiphysis; and this, although it may appear to be a much more troublesome accident, is in fact a much milder one than the other injuries at the joint.

PART 47

The treatment especially befitting each particular dislocation has been described; and it has been laid down as a rule, that immediate reduction is of the utmost advantage, owing to the rapid manner in which inflammation of the tendons supervenes. For even when the luxated parts are immediately reduced, the tendons usually become stiffened, and for a considerable time prevent extension and flexion from being performed to the ordinary extent. are to be treated in a similar way, whether the extremity of the articulating bone be snapped off, whether the bones be separated, or whether they be dislocated; for they are all to be treated with plenty of bandages, compresses, and cerate, like other fractures. The position of the joint in all these cases should be the same, as when a fractured arm or forearm has been bound up. For this is the most common position in all dislocations, displacements, and fractures; and it is the most convenient for the subsequent movements, whether of extension or flexion, as being the intermediate stage between both. And this is the position in which the patient can most conveniently carry or suspend his arm in a sling. And besides, if the joint is to be stiffened by callus, it were better that this should not take place when the arm is extended, for this position will be a great impediment and little advantage; if the arm be wholly bent, it will be more useful; but it will be much more convenient to have the joint in the intermediate position when it becomes ankylosed. So much with regard to position.

PART 48

In bandaging, the head of the first bandage should be placed at the seat of the injury, whether it be a case of fracture, of dislocation, or of diastasis (separation?), and the first turns should be made there, and the bandages should be applied most firmly at that place, and less so on either side. The bandaging should comprehend both the arm and the forearm, and on both should be to a much greater extent than most physicians apply it, so that the swelling may be expelled from the seat of the injury to either side. And point of the forearm should be comprehended in the bandaging, whether the injury be in that place or not, in order that the swelling may not collect there. In applying bandages, we must avoid as much as possible accumulating many turns of the bandage at the bend of the arm. For the principal compression should be at the seat of the injury, and the same rules are to be observed, and at the same periods, with regard to compression and relaxation, as formerly described respecting the treatment of broken bones; and the bandages should be renewed every third day; and they should appear loose on the third day, as in the other case. And splints should be applied at the proper time (for there is nothing unsuitable in them, whether the bones be fractured or not, provided there is no fever); they should be particularly loose, whether applied to the arm or the forearm, but they must not be thick. It is necessary that they should be of unequal size, and that the one should ride over the other, whenever from the flexion it is judged proper. And the application of the compresses should be regulated in the same manner as has been stated with regard to the splints; and they should be put on in a somewhat more bulky form at the seat of the injury. The periods are to be estimated from the inflammation, and from what has been written on them above.

www.ReadHowYouWant.com

You can buy our **Large Type** and **EasyRead** books from our www.ReadHowYouWant.com website, from websites like Amazon.com and through your UK and North American bookshop.

EasyRead books are designed to make your reading easy and enjoyable. **EasyRead** books are published in different font sizes, so you can select the font size best for you.

EasyRead is for people with normal eyesight who want books in an easy-to-read format.

EasyRead Comfort is for people who find reading small print tiring but do not need large print.

EasyRead Large is for people who find it easier to read larger print.

EasyRead Large Bold is for people with retinal problems who need to read high contrast text.

EasyRead Super Large is for people who require large and dense format, available in 18pt, 20pt and 24pt.

The **EasyRead** font, character, word and line spacing have all been set to make it as easy as possible both to recognize a word, and to run your eye along a line of text without losing your place. We split as few words as possible at line ends, as split words make reading harder and can be annoying. For out-of-copyright books, words have been changed to modern spelling (where the sense is not affected), and the original hyphenation of compound words has been retained where this improves word recognition or sense.

With most things you buy, you get a choice, and you can choose the make and model that suits best. There is a big exception – books. You don't get to choose a format that is easy for you to read – you have to read the format the publisher selects.

This **"One Size Fits All"** paradigm **no longer** need apply to books.

At www.ReadHowYouWant.com, you can order a book just as you want it, so you can read it easily. You can choose nearly any format, and at a surprisingly low cost, because of a technical breakthrough that allows us to typeset an individual book automatically, print and bind the book and have it quickly sent directly to you.

You can have your book in **Talking Book** formats **(DAISY or MP3)** or as an **E-book** or in **Braille**.

We have developed totally new visual formats which we hope will help people with **dyslexia** and other print reading disabilities. Look at www.ReadHowYouWant.com for more information.

Good news for publishers and authors. There is a big market for large type, personalized and accessible format books. We can help publishers and authors find new market opportunities for their books, and selling your book through www.ReadHowYouWant.com is easy – we do the work for you. Contact us on info@ReadHowYouWant.com.

Made in United States
Troutdale, OR
11/03/2026

56845131R00062